"A journey of a thousand miles begins with a single step."

– Lao-tzu

Every effort has been made to ensure that the information contained in this book is complete and accurate. However, the author is not engaged in rendering professional advice or services to the individual reader. The author has no formal medical training. The ideas, procedures, and suggestions contained in this book are not intended as a substitute for consulting with your physician and other healthcare workers. All matters regarding health require medical supervision. Neither the author nor publisher shall be liable or responsible for any loss, injury, or damage allegedly arising from any information or suggestion in this book. Also, the information in this book may not apply to all patients in that every transplant center follows its own operating procedures and uses different equipment and supplies.

Please visit our Web site at www.BMTresources.org for additional information and support. If you have any questions, suggestions, or comments about this book you can e-mail them to: contact@bmtresources.org

A portion of the proceeds from the sale of this book will be donated to The Bone Marrow Foundation to help patients in need of financial assistance for their transplants.

Table of Contents

Introduction

This book has been written with one objective in mind: To help patients who have decided to have an autologous peripheral blood stem cell transplant (PBSCT) or bone marrow transplant (BMT) get through their procedures with flying colors.

I'm Mark Patton, the most transplanted person in the world. I've had two bone marrow transplants and three stem cell transplants over the past 14 years to treat my multiple myeloma (a bone marrow cancer).

My wife Mary Grace, (M.G.), and I want to share our knowledge with transplant patients, caregivers, family members, and friends. You can avoid the pitfalls and learn from my mistakes. I may not know much, but I know transplants.

These 140 invaluable tips will help anyone, with any disease, whose treatment plan includes high-dose chemotherapy and/or radiation and transplantation. The tips provide practical, real-world information to make each day of your treatment and recovery as pleasant and problem free as possible.

The guide does not cover the highly technical aspects of these procedures. There are many books on the market that have already done that. (Please refer to the Transplant Resource Directory at the back of this book to find some of them.)

The transplant process has roughly seven phases:

1. Determining if you are a transplant candidate
2. Deciding the treatment that's best for you
3. Selecting a transplant center
4. Preparing for your transplant
5. Doing Your Transplant
6. Recovering from your chemotherapy and/or radiation
7. Maintaining your health post-transplant

We've tried to make our Transplant Resource Directory in Chapter 16 the most comprehensive ever compiled for BMTs and PBSCTs. You'll find it extremely useful.

I don't know why I've been so blessed to survive for so long. Perhaps it's to help other patients learn about the proven benefits of these miraculous procedures. To that end, I've written this book.

Let's take a few deep breaths, relax, and get started. Remember these three pieces of advice: Keep a smile on your face; keep your hospital gown tied in back; and believe in yourself. See you in remission.

Mark Patton
The World's Most Transplanted Person

Dedication

I was 41 when my multiple myeloma was diagnosed.

Early in the going, Mary Grace went in to be tested to see if
she could donate platelets to me when I needed them.
Unbelievably, her blood tests revealed she also had cancer,
chronic lymphocytic leukemia or CLL. That news, of course,
was devastating. I was at a loss.

Mary Grace never missed a beat, however. She said, "We'll get
you through your treatment, and then see about me." It was
the single most courageous act I've ever witnessed. I've
dedicated this book and my life to her.

We struck a bargain way back then. I would stay alive so I
could take care of her when she started treatment. She would
stay alive to take care of me. Sounds crazy, but it's worked for
us for the last 14 years. To date, M.G. has never had to do any
treatment for her CLL.

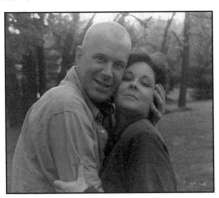

*When the night has come and the land is dark
and the moon is the only light we'll see.
No I won't be afraid, no I won't be afraid
Just as long as you stand, stand by me.*
- Ben E. King, Jerry Lieber, Mike Stoller

Chapter 1

Determining If You Are a Transplant Candidate

Incredibly, research indicates there could now be millions of bone marrow transplant (BMT) and peripheral blood stem cell transplant (PBSCT) candidates in the U.S. That's right, millions.

Clinical trials using transplants and chemotherapy and/or radiation have been conducted for the following types of cancer: esophageal; colon; rectal; pancreatic; lung and bronchial; bones & joint; melanoma; breast; uterine; ovarian; prostate; testicular; kidney; brain; lymphoma; multiple myeloma; and leukemia.

Diseases that have also had clinical trials include: many anemias; lupus; Chron's disease; systemic sclerosis; AIDS-related lymphoma; multiple sclerosis; rheumatoid arthritis; HIV; and many, many others.

Tip #1 Take advantage of the National Cancer Institute's Web site to review clinical trials that have been conducted for your type of cancer or disease. Their address is www.nci.nih.gov. Click on the *Clinical Trials* tab. You can also type *stem cell transplants* in the *search box* and pull up some wonderful information.

Tip #2 Refer to Chapter 16 for an association that can offer transplant information. (i.e. Lupus Foundation of America, American Diabetes Association, etc.)

Tip #3 You can also try to find support this way. In the *search box* of your Browser, type the name of your disease and the word *association* (i.e. multiple myeloma + association). This will normally find a resource for you.

Tip #4 Check out the National Marrow Donor Program's site at www.marrow.org. They list over 70 diseases treatable with transplants. Click on the *About NMDP* button to see the chart.

Tip #5 Several of the major transplant centers offer well over 100 clinical trials. Research trials by specific center on the National Marrow Donor Program site. The URL is www.marrow.org.

Tip #6 Don't have access to the Internet? Go to the library and ask for assistance. They'll be glad to help.

Tip #7 The American Cancer Society (www.cancer.org) offers a tool on their Web site to assist you in determining your treatment options. The tool, NexProfiler from NexCura, is a self-administered questionnaire that takes about 10 minutes to complete.

Tip #8 A number of associations and organizations can put you in touch with a survivor of your disease who has been through a transplant. You can find many of these associations in the Transplant Resource Directory.

Tip #9 One of the best places to chat with survivors is the Association of Cancer Online Resources site (www.acor.org). They have over 130 communities by specific type of disease. You can get answers to almost all your questions. They even have a *BMT Talk* group.

Tip #10 Take things you read in these online communities with a grain of salt. With so much information available today, there's a tendency for patients to jump from one treatment of the day to the next. A treatment that worked for someone else may not work for you and vice versa.

Tip #11 Try to meet with a doctor who specializes in your disease. Specialists are in a much better position to tell you if a transplant is right for you.

Bonus Tip: You may decide you don't want to undertake a transplant at this time. However, you should still see if it makes sense to collect your marrow or stem cells for a BMT or PBSCT in the future. I used stem cells that were collected and frozen in 1995 for my last transplant in February 2003. It's easier to do all these wild and crazy things when you're younger and healthier. (Be advised, though, some insurance companies will not pay for harvests or collections if a transplant date has not been set.)

Chapter 2

Some Background Information on Transplants

BMTs and PBSCTs are proven, highly effective treatments for curing certain diseases and greatly extending the lives of countless thousands of patients. The first successful allogeneic BMT (using donor marrow) was done in 1957 in Cooperstown, New York. The first successful autologous BMT (using the patient's own marrow) took place in France in 1968. Today, there are more than 50,000 transplants being done each year.

There are three main types of transplants:
- Autologous - the patient uses his or her own cells or marrow
- Allogeneic - the patient uses a donor's cells or marrow
- Syngeneic - the patient uses cells or marrow from an identical twin

Tip #12 The National Cancer Institute's Web site offers a free, online brochure that provides excellent information in a simple Question & Answer format for BMTs and PBSCTs. Go to www.nci.nih.gov and click on NCI Publications.

Tip #13 The Bone Marrow Foundation offers two free booklets on transplantation, one for allogeneic transplants and the other for autologous transplants.

You can read them online or have them send you the brochures. (www.bonemarrow.org)

Tip #14 MEDLINEplus (www.medlineplus.org) has more than 30 articles on BMTs and PBSCTs. Click on *Health Topics*, click on *Procedures and Therapies*, and select *Bone Marrow Transplantation.*

Tip #15 Stem cells used in BMTs and PBSCTs are adult stem cells, not to be confused with embryonic stem cells. Occasionally, stem cells from umbilical cords are used in transplants, but again, these are not the controversial embryonic stem cells.

Tip #16 Transplants are not without risk. Discuss the risks and benefits with your physician and survivors. Remember, if they weren't relatively safe procedures, however, there wouldn't be 50,000 done each year.

Bonus Tip: Ask your doctor if you're a candidate for a *mini-transplant*. A *mini* uses a less toxic, lower dose of chemotherapy. It is often used for older patients and those who have other health complications. These procedures are also referred to as *non-myeloablative* or *reduced-intensity* transplants.

Find out more about these procedures by visiting www.lymphomation.org, www.ibmtindy.com, or www.clinicaltrials.gov.

Chapter 3

Deciding the Treatment that's Best for You

(Clinical Trials vs. Individualized Treatment)

Your doctor will tell you if he or she thinks you'd benefit more from being in a clinical trial or whether you should have a treatment plan individualized for you. This decision is based on your age, overall health, disease status, and prior treatments.

Many clinical trials are designed for patients who have relapsed (called refractory disease) or who have failed to respond significantly to prior treatments. Often the trials will use a drug that has been fast-tracked by the FDA for patients who have no other options.

This is an all-important point in the process and one that requires you to ask a million questions and really do your homework. The more you believe in your treatment and your physician, the better you'll do. Honestly.

Tip #17 You always have the right to drop out of a clinical trial if the side effects become too severe. I've bailed out of two.

Tip #18 Be advised, the company sponsoring the trial can drop you if they so choose. This will happen if you're not responding sufficiently to the treatment (a somewhat arbitrary judgment call on occasion). Clarify this in advance.

Tip #19 Your doc can remove you from a protocol if he or she feels another course of action will get better results. I went off trial to do four sessions of TBI (total body irradiation) to further reduce my disease burden.

Tip #20 Almost all the costs of participating in a clinical trial are paid for by the sponsoring company. Read the trial paperwork thoroughly to see if there are any costs, in any event, that might not be covered. Then you can see if your insurance covers those costs.

Tip #21 Clinical trials are customarily divided into two groups: those who receive the new drug, or combination of drugs and treatment; and those who get the standard treatment. There's no way of knowing ahead of time which group you'll be in so you may not get the new stuff.

Tip #22 Don't compare your trial or treatment with other patient's. This will lead to an endless game of second-guessing why they're doing things you're not or you're doing things they're not. Make your decision and stay the course.

Chapter 4

Selecting a Transplant Center

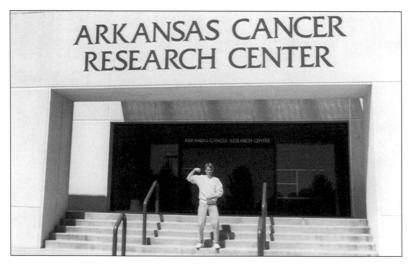

The best case situation is to have a hospital in your town or area that can do your transplant. At present, there are over 200 centers nationally.

Many patients, however, will have to travel to another city for their procedure. For example, you might want to go to a center that specializes in your type of cancer or disease. We went to the Arkansas Cancer Research Center for treatment. The center recently performed its 5,000th stem cell transplant, most of which have been done for myeloma patients.

MD Anderson Cancer Center in Houston performs over 600 blood and marrow transplants on adults and children each year, making them one of the largest and most experienced centers in the world.

Tip #23 The Fred Hutchinson Cancer Research Center (www.fhcrc.org) has a feature on its Web site entitled *How To Choose a Transplant Center*. Click on *Treatment and Patient Services*.

Tip #24 The National Marrow Donor Program (www.marrow.org) also informs visitors how to select a transplant center. Go to their site and click *Patient Resources*.

Tip #25 Another organization to visit is the Gift of Life Bone Marrow Foundation (www.bone-marrow.org). Click the *Patient* tab.

Chapter 5

Preparing for Your Transplant

Central Venous Catheters

One of the most important decisions you may have to make before having your transplant will be what type of central venous catheter (CVC) you want and where you want it placed.

Your CVC, or central line as it's also called, is a small flexible tube inserted into the large vein above your heart. Your catheter will be used to administer drugs, blood products, and sometimes nutrition. Blood samples can be taken from your line, which will save you the pain of being stuck countless times with a needle.

There are two types of catheters available: external and internal. External catheters (called Hickman's) are tunneled under your skin but the two lumens dangle on the outside of your body. Internal catheters are completely implanted under the skin. The only evidence you have one is a small bump on your chest about the size of a quarter.

Tip #26 Active people who want to bathe and swim without restriction should go for the internal catheter or port. It's nearly maintenance-free. The external (Hickman) requires more care and cleaning.

Tip #27 Think about whether you want your catheter on your left or right side. Things that can rub against your port include seatbelts and straps from bags and luggage.

If you sleep primarily on your right side, you might want to have your catheter placed on your left.

Tip #28 Internal catheters (ports) usually have one, two, or three lumens. I've had single and double. Ask your doc if he or she has any opinions on the matter.

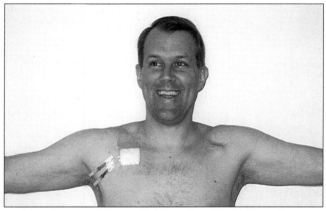

Here's me with my Quinton (on the left) and my port (barely visible on the right)

Bonus Tip: Some institutions do not give the patient a choice on the type of catheter or number of lumens. The transplant team makes those decisions.

Preconditioning Chemotherapy and/or Radiation Treatment

The type of preconditioning treatment patients receive prior to transplant varies by disease and the individual patient's needs. These treatments are designed to kill off as many cancer cells as possible.

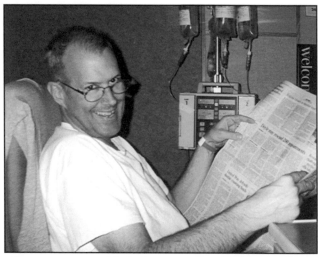

The ever-present infusion pump and bags of drugs

Tip #29 The chemo you get now can be fairly hard on you, and might require hospitalization. Ask your doctor if this step can be done on an outpatient basis.

Tip #30 Your preparative treatment is often powerful enough to make you quite tired and cause your hair to fall out. Talk it over with your physician so you're not surprised when this happens. (Refer to Chapter 8, Dealing with Hair Loss.)

Tip #31 Most treatments require you go to the hospital, clinic, or doctor's office to receive them. Others allow you to continue your normal (pretty much) daily activities. I wore a little holster with a tube of chemo under my work shirt for four days of each month for three months. No one knew I had it on. If you work outside the home, be clear on how your treatment will affect your job.

Tip #32 The more you can get involved in your own treatment, the fewer times you'll have to go to the hospital or doctor's office. You and your primary caregiver may be asked if you are capable and willing to change chemo tubing, give subcutaneous shots, flush your catheter lines, and so on. Do it if you can. It will save you a ton of time.

Stem Cell Collections

Patients doing stem cell transplants will go through a process known as stem cell apheresis to collect their cells. Lucky you, you get another catheter for apheresis.

Your second catheter will be a Quinton. It will be inserted into a vein in the other side of your chest. Don't despair. You'll only have this catheter for a few days. It's amazing how quickly and painlessly Quintons are inserted by a doctor.

Usually, you'll be given a number of injections of a drug called G-CSF, granulocyte stimulating colony factor. This drug stimulates your body into making millions of stem cells for your collection.

The collection (apheresis) will take one, two, three, or more days, depending on how many cells they can get during each session. As soon as you're finished, you can probably get rid of your Quinton catheter, although some centers leave it in until your transplant.

Tip #33 You'll probably be asked if you or your caregiver can administer the G-CSF shots. Again, if you're able, I recommend biting the bullet and doing it at home rather than visiting the doctor's office, clinic, or hospital everyday.

Tip #34 Your nurse will recommend sites for the injections. These will include the back of the upper arms, the thighs, and the stomach. Surprisingly, the stomach is no more painful that any of the other sites.

Bonus Tip: Try not to irritate your caregiver if he or she is giving you your shot. I only made that mistake one time.

Tip #35 You may get the chills while doing your collection. Apheresis can deplete your electrolytes. Chewing antacid tablets can replace some of the calcium you've lost and help stop the chills.

Tip #36 Make sure you've used the water closet before apheresis starts. One session can last two to four hours. They can stop the machine if you have to go to the bathroom, but it's an involved routine to disconnect and reconnect you.

Bone Marrow Harvests

Patients undergoing a bone marrow transplant will have their marrow harvested while under a general anesthesia (knocked-out). The doctor or technician will extract the marrow from the iliac crest, which is that hard bony area above your backside. The sternum (breastbone) is another extraction site, but rarely used for a harvest. The entire harvest can take less than 90 minutes including prep time.

Tip #37 I've had trips to the dentist that were more painful than my harvest. You may have some tenderness in the area for the next few days, but it's no big thing. My wife and I made a 12-hour car ride home the day after my harvest.

Tip #38 Enjoy a long bath or shower before your harvest because you won't be able to take one for several days afterwards.

Tip #39: Many things you'll have to do during your transplant sound kind of scary at first blush. Take it from me, they're not that bad. With the right attitude, and the right medications, you'll be just fine.

Chapter 6

Doing Your Transplant

Your Length of Stay

Congratulations! You made it through your conditioning therapy. You've also successfully navigated your bone marrow harvest or stem cell collections if you're doing an autologous transplant.

Tip #40 The length of time between your conditioning therapy and your transplant will depend on how well you've responded to the treatment and the state of your overall health. It's fairly common to go through a recovery period of several months before your transplant date. Often, you get more chemo and/or radiation just before you're transplanted.

For my third PBSCT, I was given my chemo in November and transplanted three months later in February. The lag time for my first transplant was about the same.

Tip #41 In the early days of transplants (1980s), patients were often in isolation for a month or more. Today, many procedures are being done on an outpatient basis. Ask if you're an outpatient candidate or how long you'll be incarcerated if all goes well.

Tip #42 Patients undergoing an autologous (auto) BMT or PBSCT are typically released from the hospital much sooner because they don't have to worry about graft-versus-host disease (GVHD), which can happen with allogeneic (allo) transplants.

Tip #43 Learn more about GVHD by visiting The Lymphoma & Leukemia Society's Web page at www.leukemia.org. Click on the *Glossary* button and click on the letter *G* and scroll down.

Tip #44 Allo transplant patients should ensure they know how long they will have to stay near the hospital or center. The old rule of thumb used to be 100 days.

Your Hospital Room

Your hospital room could be your home away from home for anywhere from several days to several weeks or more. Patients facing a longer stay should make their rooms as comfortable and homey as possible.

During my numerous stays over the years, I've seen patients and family members bring in computers, rocking chairs, rugs, mirrors, pictures, special blankets, CD players, DVD players, and even an artificial Christmas tree.

Tip #45 Make your room your own, but don't kill your caregivers by requesting they bring in the hot tub or big screen TV.

Tip #46 Don't like the way your furniture is arranged? Rearrange it. As long as you're not blocking access to the doors or equipment, no one should complain.

Every hospital room in the galaxy is identical. They all contain:

- Infinitely adjustable hospital bed
- Geri chair (the heaviest, ugliest recliner on the planet)
- Infusion pump (for your chemo, blood products, and meds)
- Infinitely adjustable thermostat
- TV with remote control, light switch, and nurse call button
- A tiny bathroom with an even smaller shower
- Portable commode
- Heart monitor
- Tray on wheels
- Bulletin board or marker board (optional)

Tip #47 Your bed is actually more of an amusement ride than a bed. It's very uncomfortable, but you can while away the hours playing with it, trying to find the exact right position, which you never will.

Tip #48 Don't ever try to move the Geri chair unless you've competed in Olympic weightlifting competitions.

Tip #49 Your infusion pump will be your best pal for your hospitalization. It will be by your side night and day. Don't worry if you see little air bubbles in the line. They won't hurt you.

Tip #50 The infusion pump will sound an alarm (beep) if the drip gets interrupted or the infusion is complete. Summon your nurse and she or he will come fix it.

Tip #51 You can spend most of the day and night connected to your infusion pump early in the process. Always have the nurse run the line from your IV bag to your catheter under your shirt rather than down through the neck hole. When it goes down through the neck hole, you can't take your shirt or top off without being disconnected. Putting on another shirt or taking off the one you're wearing becomes a rigmarole.

Tip #52 The nurse call button is right next to the button that turns your TV on and off. You will often push the call button by mistake. Practice saying this line, "I'm terribly sorry. I pushed the wrong button."

Tip #53 Your infusion pump will always start beeping when you're in the bathroom. It never fails.

Tip #54 The portable commode is an unpleasant concept but a necessity. There may be times when you have to use it. Your need to go can become so urgent you won't have time to unplug your pump, roll up the cord, and push the contraption into the bathroom. You have no other choice. Grin and bear it.

Tip #55 You won't cross paths with the heart monitor unless you pick up a bug. The monitor tracks your heart rate, blood pressure, and oxygen level. Being on the heart monitor will mean having to use the portable commode. You can't get very far from your bed.

Bonus Tip (Men only): Don't even think about disconnecting yourself from the heart monitor so you can go to the bathroom. I did and got a nice tongue-lashing. The nurses thought I had flat lined or something when the monitor went screwy at the nurse's station. Again, you've got to go with the flow.

Your Transplant

Your big day will arrive before you know it. Often, you're transplanted two or three days after you're admitted to the hospital and given your big blast of chemo and/or radiation. The best word to describe the actual transplant is . . . anti-climactic. This is true of both BMTs and PBSCTs.

On transplant day (Day 0), there'll be a flurry of activity as the transplant team begins getting your room ready and coordinating things with the lab technicians who will take your marrow or stem cells out of the freezer to thaw before bringing them to your room.

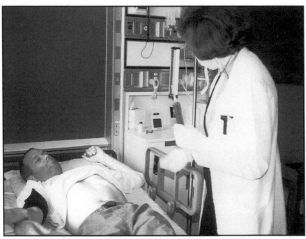

*That big syringe in the nurse's hand
holds my bone marrow.*

For those doing a BMT, the marrow comes to your room in several large syringes. Bone marrow is a deep purple color. The transplant nurse then injects (pushes) the marrow into your central line (catheter) over a period of about five minutes per syringe.

For those doing a PBSCT, the stem cells are contained in small IV bags. They are more of a pale yellow color and look somewhat like platelets. The transplant nurse or doctor hangs the bags from your IV pole and they drip into your central line. It takes about 20 to 30 minutes per bag. The number of bags infused (total volume) is different for each patient.

See, all that worrying for nothing. It's simple and painless.

Tip #56 Right after a BMT, your urine can turn kind of a deep purple color for a little while. It's perfectly normal but startling if you haven't been told.

Tip #57 Don't get too caught up in the hubbub going on in your room with all the preparations. Just relax and think about the miracle you're participating in. Many transplant patients refer to the day as their second birthday.

Chapter 7

Recovering from Your Chemotherapy and/or Radiation

The toughest part of the entire process is recovering from the effects of the treatment you've been given to prepare you for your transplant. By the time your transplant rolls around, there's an excellent chance you've already been through high-dose chemotherapy, radiation treatments, or both. If so, you know the drill.

Surviving Neutropenia

Understanding Your Complete Blood Count is a publication available from the National Institutes of Health. It defines white blood cells, neutrophils, and neutropenia in the following manner:

"White blood cells – These cells are the mobile units of the body's infection-fighting system. White blood cells travel in the bloodstream to areas of infection and destroy the responsible bacteria.

Neutrophils are the most numerous white blood cells. They make up about 56 percent of white blood cells. Neutrophils are the "soldiers" that fight infection.

The normal neutrophil count is 2,500 - 6,000. When you have 1,000 or fewer neutrophils, your risk of infection is increased. When your ANC (absolute neutrophil count) is lower than 500, you're at risk of getting a serious infection. This condition is called neutropenia."

Making it through neutropenia without getting sick will be your biggest transplant challenge. It will take several weeks or months for your counts to rise to the point where the risk of infection isn't so great. These tips will help you avoid running into complications. Some I researched, others I learned the hard way.

There are seven essentials for sailing through neutropenia:

1. Maintaining good hygiene
2. Eating properly
3. Drinking plenty of fluids
4. Taking your medicine
5. Staying active
6. Keeping a positive attitude
7. Taking precautions against infection

Tip #58 The Oncology Nursing Society's Web site has good information about dealing with neutropenia and other major cancer treatment symptoms. The can be found at www.cancersymptoms.org.

Tip #59 Visit the American Cancer Society's Web page or call them (the number is in the Transplant Resource Directory). Request a copy of their booklet *Fever and Neutropenia Guidelines.* You can also download the booklet if you prefer. It's a wonderful read for neutropenics who want to stay healthy.

Tip #60 You shouldn't have to ask when you become neutropenic, you should be told when the day comes so you can be on guard. Many hospitals provide a marker board in your room and the nurses will post your counts daily. You'll get a strong sense of progress watching your blood counts climb.

Maintaining Good Hygiene

Personal hygiene is extremely important while your immune system is compromised (neutropenic). It can be a struggle, but keep up your routine of oral care and bathing to prevent problems.

Tip #61 Showering is a challenge especially if your catheter is accessed (your getting an infusion at the time). Even if you're not being infused, the tubing from your port hangs down about six inches. You have to assume a crazy, unnatural stance in the shower as to not get your port and bandaging wet.

Tip #62 Ask your nurse if you can take a bath if that's your preference. Some hospitals can accommodate you.

Tip #63 Should you not be up to showering or a conventional bath, the nurse might be able to supply you with disposable wash clothes that heat up in a microwave. You can use them on your body and hair. I tried them once and liked them. They were no muss, no fuss and did a good job.

Tip #64 Any time you aren't receiving an infusion is a good time to jump in the shower. You can work with the nurse to plan your shower or bath around your infusions. Also, when the time comes to change the needle in your catheter (every few days) take advantage of your freedom to clean up.

Tip #65 Don't skip washing. If you can't do it alone, and you have no caregiver to assist you, tell the nurse you need help. Swallow your shyness and wash daily.

Tip #66 Another area of critical importance is oral care. Chemo and radiation can interfere (temporarily) with your saliva glands. The result is dry mouth. A dry mouth is the perfect environment for breeding bacteria and fungi. You should get a saline solution (saltwater) to use everyday to brush your teeth and gargle.

Tip #67 You'll also get a spongy toothbrush to use. Having low platelets while you're neutropenic can cause your gums to bleed. This little brush will reduce the chance of bleeding.

Bonus Tip: A buildup on your tongue that looks a bit like fur and is yellowish is a sign you're developing a fungal infection (thrush). Tell your nurse immediately so you can get the proper medication to deal with it before it gets a head of steam.

Tip #68 I recommend saliva pills for dry mouth. You can find them at any drug store. Hard candy works, too, but it's tough on your teeth unless it's sugar free.

Tip #69 Your high-dose chemo and radiation can cause your skin to become very dry and crack. Cracked skin is an open door for bacteria. Rub yourself down with a body or skin lotion. If you have a willing caregiver, this can be a nice, relaxing part of your day.

Tip #70 I suggest you stay away from the perfumed or heavily scented lotions. You're going to be feeling queasy to begin with and this type of smell may make you good and nauseous. Inexpensive lotions work just as well as the expensive kind.

Tip #71 Chemo can produce a bit of a burning sensation when it passes from your body. Diarrhea is a common side effect. If you begin to have a sensitivity problem, you should get some of those flushable wipes to soothe your woes.

Tip #72 A final piece of advice in this area. Don't let your lips get cracked and start bleeding. Slather on your favorite lip balm several times a day.

Eating Properly

Proper nutrition during neutropenia is comprised of two parts: eating enough and eating the right things. Your recovery can be delayed significantly by not paying attention to both parts of this equation.

Eating enough is a problem because of the nauseous feeling brought on by your treatment. You won't feel like eating at all. The sick-to-your-stomach feeling can last for weeks sometimes.

Eating the wrong things can really move you from the frying pan to the fire should you wind up with food poisoning or ingesting other bacteria. Avoid questionably prepared and raw foods at all costs.

Tip #73 The American Cancer Society has some very good pages on their Web site under the heading *When Treatment Causes Eating Problems.* These pages also contain some recipes you might find useful.

Tip #74 Transplant centers have outstanding dietitians on staff. Spend as much time as you need talking to the dietitian to work out a menu that includes the kinds of food you can get down and keep down.

Tip #75 Go for bland, soft foods. Try eggs, potatoes, puddings, soups, pancakes, waffles, gelatins, ice cream, milk shakes, and cereals. Eat as much as you can, even if it's a real struggle. Those patients who can't eat enough wind up getting their nutrition by IV.

Tip #76 In the event you simply can't eat a lot or you develop mouth or throat problems like mucousitis, you can ask for a liquid nutritional supplement such as Boost or Ensure. Anything to pack in the calories.

Tip #77 Don't be shy about requesting an anti-nausea drug (also called an antiemetic) before your meal time. They can settle your stomach and allow you to get more down and keep it down.

Tip #78 Count on every single meal you're served being interrupted. People will show up to take your vitals, weigh you, take you to x-ray, conduct rounds, find out what you want at your next meal, offer you spiritual guidance, give you your medications, change your bedding, change your catheter lines, and subject you to other indignities. Have someone guard your meal tray should you have to leave the room. Ask, politely, if folks can come back at another time.

Tip #79 We all have our comfort foods. You may have foods that will be more palatable than others. My wife would bring in mashed potatoes, rice, pudding, and milk shakes when it was difficult for me to face the hospital food. I encourage you to do the same if nutrition is becoming a problem. Check with your team to ensure none of the foods brought in are on the *forbidden list.*

Drinking Plenty of Fluids

Fluids play a critical role in recovery from chemo and/or radiation. Chemo can dry you out so much you may peel from head to toe. The National Institutes of Health (NIH) publishes a booklet entitled *Eating Hints for Cancer Patients.* The recommendation in this book is to drink 6 to 8 cups (48 to 64 ounces) of liquids per day. Here are a few drinks and liquids you can put into the mix:

- water
- carbonated soft drinks (lemon-lime)
- lemonade
- juices (orange, cranberry, grape, etc.)
- Gatorade
- flavored vitamin waters
- broth
- Popsicles
- teas
- fruit-flavored drinks
- ice chips

Tip #80 You may want to avoid drinks that are too acidic (like citrus juices) if you're having trouble with your stomach.

Tip #81 Your nurses will constantly offer to bring fresh cups of water. Never pass up the chance to get one, especially at night. There's nothing worse in the whole world than waking up with cotton-mouth and nothing to drink.

Taking Your Medicine

Your transplant medications (meds) come in two kinds; the kind you'll be given and the kind you're going to have to ask for. The list below encompasses most of the meds you'll need and want.

Chemoprotectants

This is a relatively new class of drug. Amifostine (or Eythol) can protect both your liver and your digestive system from the harsh side effects of chemo when given in advance. It will reduce your chance of developing mucousitis, a painful mouth and throat condition, which makes it very difficult to swallow.

Tip #82 Bring this medication up in discussion with your doc if he or she doesn't bring it up first.

Antiemetics

Chemo and radiation affect different people in different ways. Some don't have major reactions. Others get sicker than dogs. All told, I've been through nine rounds of high-dose chemo and four sessions of total body irradiation (radiation). I relied quite a bit on antiemetics to help me through.

Tip #83 When you feel sick to your stomach and throw up, it will only make you feel sicker and want to throw up more. Stay out of this cycle by taking some antiemetics as soon as you start to feel queasy.

Tip #84 Some of these drugs come in pill and liquid form. If you feel yourself becoming nauseous very rapidly, tell your nurse you want a liquid dose put directly into your central line (catheter). It's known as an *IV push*.

Sleepers

You will never get a good night sleep in a hospital. Nurses, technicians, doctors, housekeeping staff, and a host of others will enter your room all night to do various necessary and unnecessary things. Sleep deprivation can make you irritable and cranky, and you already have enough problems so you don't want that. You need your beauty rest to recover.

Tip #85 I avoided taking sleeping pills until my last two hospital stays. I wish I had smartened up sooner. Don't be hesitant to try them should you feel you're becoming sleep deprived and grouchy.

Tip #86 Nurses will not administer sleepers after 3:00 a.m. It makes the patient too groggy the next day. Don't wait too long if you want one.

Bonus Tip: Your doctor will have given the staff on your transplant floor a list of drugs you are preapproved to take. Your nurse will have to get an OK from your doc to give you any med not on the preapproved list.

Review your preapproved list of medications before you check into the hospital.

Antifungals
You can develop fungal infections in your mouth (thrush) and in your fingernails and toenails while your immune system is weakened.

Tip #87 Again, if you notice a coating on your tongue (a furry or hairy appearance), bring it to your nurse's attention. Fingernail and toenail infections come in all colors and sizes. I had one in a thumbnail that started off emerald green. Show anything suspicious to your healthcare providers.

Tip #88 Thrush infections can be quite painful. To alleviate the pain, you can ask your nurse for a solution you can swish around in your mouth and spit out.

Tip #89 Some oral, liquid medications are *swish and spits* and others are *swish and swallows*. Read the label and don't swallow if you should be spitting.

Antibiotics
These drugs kill bacteria but not viruses. Bacterial infections of the ear, bladder, kidneys, and sinuses are treated with antibiotics. Many pneumonias and strep throat are also treated with these medications.

Tip #90 Nip any and all problems you begin to develop in the bud. Your body temperature is an excellent indicator of a bacterial infection. A temp of around 100 degrees F or higher means something's cooking and needs to be addressed.

Antivirals

The webMDHealth's Web site (www.webmd.com) describes antivirals this way: "Antivirals are drugs used to treat viral infections just as antibiotics are used to treat bacterial infections. The main practical difference is that antivirals for herpes and other forms of viruses don't kill the virus and wipe out the infection. These antivirals inhibit the virus' replication process."

Most upper respiratory infections (URIs) and the shingles are viruses.

Tip #91 A rash that appears as a belt around your waist or appears on your face could be the shingles. Point out anything suspicious like this to your nurse. The shingles can be very bothersome and last a very long time.

Pain Medications

Some patients enter the BMT or PBSCT process in relatively good health, other than their disease. Other patients are not so fortunate. Those that have multiple myeloma can have compression fractures and broken bones by the time they are diagnosed and treatment commences.

Also, patients can be in pain from other diseases or conditions and the transplant process may exacerbate those problems. I had bad back pain during my last transplant, probably from a compression fracture.

The long and the short of it is, if you're in pain, you probably don't have to be. Tell your doc what's ailing you and he or she can prescribe something to help.

Tip #92 Some patients have an unrealistic fear about becoming addicted to pain pills. Overall, that possibility is pretty remote. Taking some narcotics while your hospitalized, which will allow you to sleep and to get up and around, is just part of the recovery process for many.

Tip #93 I would like to stress the point that there is nothing painful about a BMT or PBSCT itself. Discomfort comes form the conditions that arise as the result of chemo and radiation treatment.

Tip #94 Take all of your meds when they are given to you while you're in the hospital. Don't let them stack up. Skipping your medications will delay your recovery or, worse yet, you'll wind up with some other problem that you could have avoided. You may not feel like doing it, but hold your nose and keep choking them down.

Tip #95 You can put your pills in foods like applesauce, yogurt, or pudding if it helps you get them down. Your nurse can provide other pill-taking tips.

Pre-Medications

Pre-meds are administered prior to a test or procedure to make you more comfortable and lessen your anxiety. A lot of folks really dislike the idea of being placed inside a CAT scan machine or an MRI tube. If you feel like you could benefit from pre-meds, your nurse will offer some suggestions.

Tip #96 Make sure if you request a pre-med before your test or procedure that it's given to you so that it has enough time to work.

Tip #97 Oftentimes, patients given pre-medications will not be able to drive home. Have a caregiver drive or help you home.

Bonus Tip: Patients with blood and marrow cancers often have to undergo bone marrow biopsies and aspirations. These procedures can be painful if done incorrectly. I've probably done three or four dozen. The key to a painless procedure is a good strong pre-med cocktail (i.e. versid and Demerol), lots of topical anesthesia (i.e. lidicane) and a doctor, P.A., N.P. or technician who takes plenty of time. Anyone who says you don't need a pre-med prior to a biopsy has never had one.

Staying Active

Feeling lousy tends to make you want to lie around in bed watching TV and drooling. Resist this urge. Patients who keep themselves moving and exercising do much better and recover faster than those who don't.

The big social event for most folks is walking the halls with their IV poles and pumps rolling along beside them. Those who are a bit unsteady on their feet can ask a nurse or caregiver to walk with them. Even if you can just make it 20 or 30 feet on your first outing, it's better than being on your backside in bed thinking poor, poor pitiful me.

Your team takes exercising seriously. I've seen instances where they've gone into patients' rooms and literally hoisted them out of bed to get them moving.

Tip #98 Your chemo kills off a big percentage of your red blood cells which is normal. Red blood cells carry oxygen to your organs and brain. Standing up too quickly when your red count is low can make you very dizzy and faint. Rise slowly until you have your sea legs.

Tip #99 Don't overdo things, it's not a competition. One elderly gent on our floor heard that 82 laps amounted to one mile. He made his mile but went into some kind of cardiac arrhythmia shortly thereafter. All things in moderation.

Keeping a Positive Attitude

Years back, there was a story about a man who was diagnosed with a fatal disease. He began watching funny movies all day everyday. He actually laughed himself into remission. I tend to believe this story. You can never underestimate the power of your mind.

Some patients bring in their briefcases and notebook computers and continue to work while they are hospitalized. Others bring in crafts or hobbies to keep themselves occupied and entertained. Still others read inspirational books and affirmations. I listened to my favorite music, watched old movies, read, and worked a little crossword puzzle game.

Tip #100 I think the work thing is great, if you're up to it, and only if you truly enjoy your work.

Tip #101 Many transplant floors have video players and movies you can watch. See if your floor does.

Tip #102 Avoid family members and friends who are down-in-the-mouth. Some people have an unfathomable need to tell cancer patients about friends who didn't do well with their disease.

Taking Precautions Against Infection

The American Cancer Society publishes and distributes a *Fever and Neutropenia Treatment Guidelines* booklet. It can be downloaded from their site (www.cancer.org), or call them to get a hard copy.

A section of this booklet is entitled, *How To Reduce Your Risk of Infection.* It provides excellent advice on avoiding infections. Infections that occur while you're neutropenic are, as a rule, the single biggest complication encountered in the transplant process. I highly recommend reading this booklet.

These are just a few of the suggestions:

- Avoid large crowds of people and anyone with a cold, flu, or other infection
- Keep your body clean by bathing each day and washing your hands after using the bathroom
- Wash your hands before eating
- Don't keep fresh flowers or live plants in your room
- Don't clean up droppings from pets; let someone else do this for you
- Use hot water to clean your dishes
- Don't share bath towels or drinking glasses with others

You'll also find a list of foods you shouldn't eat and guidelines for fluid consumption.

Tip #103 Let everyone who is coming to visit know about the *No flowers/No plants Rule*. We had nurses crack open the door, show us beautiful flowers and plants, and tell us they'd be waiting outside for my wife to lug home at the end of the day. We gave many arrangements away to nurses, aides, and technicians.

Tip #104 Don't expect your caregiver to take the flowers and plants home at the end of the day. They'll have plenty of other things to tote.

Tip #105 Washing your hands constantly throughout the day can make them raw. If you can afford it, bring in a bottle of liquid hand sanitizer. These products kill germs and some even have moisturizers in them.

Tip #106 This is a tough one. Doctors and other healthcare providers who come into your room are supposed to wash their hands before examining or touching you. If you don't see them do it, you can ask them to do it. As you can imagine, this is a little touchy.

Tip #107 You'll be able to go out in public as your counts recover. This, however, doesn't mean you're ready to throw caution to the wind. Again, avoid large crowds, those who are obviously ill, and dirty restaurants and restrooms.

Bonus Tip: You may also want to skip the family and friend parties where there will be a boatload of kids and germs. I was suckered in on this one twice.

Chapter 8

Dealing with Hair Loss

Losing one's locks from chemo or radiation is a traumatic event for many. Women struggle with this side-effect much more than men. Those who have already had plenty of treatment prior to their transplant are used to this glitch.

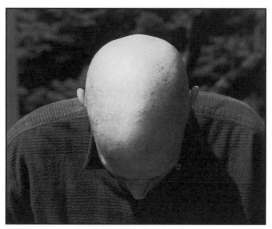

Now that's bald!

For those who have not yet experienced sudden hair loss, take heart. There are scads of products and resources out there to help you through this temporary, cue ball situation.

Personally, my first balding was hard. The next six or seven were no big deal. Fortunately, the clean head look is in right now for men. I got a great ball cap from friends that says, "Wish you were hair."

So don't fret. You'll be through it in no time and back to your gorgeous self.

Tip #108 Undergoing heavy-duty treatment can make all the hair on your body fall out. That's all your hair, everywhere. Available accessories, in addition to wigs and toupees, include eyebrows and eyelashes. They got you covered.

Tip #109 Go to the Transplant Resource Directory and read about two companies that have products for dealing with hair loss; Headcovers Unlimited and tlc Catalog.

Tip #110 You will hear stories of folks who went through treatment and never lost a strand of hair. Your doctor can give you the straight scoop on whether you'll be lockless or not. My doc was right almost to the day. Don't set yourself up for an unnecessary fall.

Tip #111 I recommend cutting your hair very short before it starts to come out. Then, you can just rub a wash cloth over your dome to remove it when the time is right. It beats finding hair all over your bed and room.

Tip #112 Visit the ACS Web site for a list of things to do for hair loss. You'll learn a good deal about the subject. You can also visit your local office.

Tip #113 Scarves and bandannas trap less heat than hats or wigs. Bandannas were my preference. If you're a guy and you think someone might laugh at you, buy your bandanna, skull cap, or *do-rag* from Harley-Davidson.

Tip #114 Almost everyone will need an all cotton, super comfortable cap to sleep in during the winter. M.G. found a small, lightweight stocking cap that was perfect.

Bonus Tip: It's pretty common for someone's hair to come back in a different color and texture. A friend whose hair was straight and brunette had her hair grow out auburn and curly. Mine went from mostly gray to mostly dark brown.

Tip #115 Go to the Web site www.scrubs.com for a dazzling array of scrub caps and head covers. Their products will let you express your individuality and personal style.

Chapter 9

The Input/Output Game

The Input/Output Game is one of the fun activities you can look forward to when you do your transplant. In short, everything you take in (eat and drink) and everything you put out (you get the idea) will be measured.

This lets your doctor know your insides are still working fine and nothing has shutdown because of your treatment.

Your nurse, dietitian, or other staff member will ask you everyday about the things you've had to drink and eat. Then, they can estimate the total number of fluid ounces and calories you've consumed.

They can calculate the calories by looking at how much of each meal you've eaten or not eaten.

Men use a plastic urinal to collect their pee. It's about the size of a quart of milk. Women use a plastic device that looks like an upside-down cowboy hat. It hangs down inside the toilet. You pour the pee from the hat into a urinal.

You will also be asked if you've moved your bowels each day. If not, you can be given a stool softener or laxative or both.

Tip #116 A good nurse will come in many times a shift to record your output and empty your urinal. A not so good nurse will ignore your urinal, wait for you to empty it, and take your word for the volume. Resist the temptation to cheat the system by skipping the collection. You'll wind up cheating yourself.

Tip #117 The men's urinal has a lid that's attached by a plastic strap. You have to try and take care of business with one hand while holding the handle of the jug and pushing the top back with your thumb. More than once, my top flipped back over the opening mid-stream with very unpleasant results. My solution was to cut the top off and see who yelled at me. No one ever did.

The Input/Output Game takes an interesting turn if you catch a bug. Bug catchers have to save some of their stool. For that, everybody uses the cowboy hat. By collecting a stool sample, a culture can be done to help determine the exact bug that's climbed onboard so it can be treated. Men seem to have more of a problem than women collecting stool samples. Men, buck up and do what you gotta do.

Chapter 10

Taking Care of Your Healthcare Providers

Someone once said it takes a village to raise a child. Well, if that's true, it takes a metropolis to get a patient through a BMT or PBSCT.

First come your primary physicians; oncologists, internists, G.P.s, and the like. Then, there are the secondary docs who are needed when you run into trouble. During my transplants, I crossed paths with ENT docs, cardiologists, infectious disease docs, gastroenterologists, rhuematologists, and radiologists, to name just a few.

Next, in no particular order, you could have: physician's assistants, nurse practitioners, RNs, LPNs, nurse's aides, technicians, housekeepers, chaplains, transportation people, dietitians, and meal service staff.

Each of these people is a trained professional and deserves your respect. They are all helping to facilitate your transplant procedure. As they sing in the hit show *Chicago*, "You be good to mama and mama will be good to you."

Tip #118 Healthcare workers have very stressful jobs. Like anyone else, they like treats and surprises. One night, M.G. bought pizzas for all the nurses on the night shift. No matter what treat you offer, it will be appreciated and remembered.

Tip #119 Try to think ahead to make your nurse's job easier. Don't let her or him walk out of your room and then ring the call button two seconds later asking for something.

Bonus Tip: Keep the whining to an absolute minimum. They've heard it all before and it puts you in a bad light.

Chapter 11

Caring for Your Caregiver

Most transplant patients will have one or more family members and friends who will help them on their journey. I've seen a few poor souls who seemed to be going it alone. I don't know how they managed.

Your primary caregiver will be your lifeline throughout your PBSCT or BMT. Never forget, the process will be very hard on your caregiver as well. A typical day for M.G. during my transplants looked something like this:

5:30 a.m. - Up and at 'em

6:00 a.m. - Finish doing laundry from night before

6:30 a.m. - Work from home as financial consultant

9:30 a.m. - Leave for hospital

10:00 a.m. - Pick up lunch or stuff to make lunch

10:30 a.m. - Arrive at hospital and put away laundry and food

11:00 a.m. - Sit in uncomfortable chair and keep grumpy patient happy

12:00 p.m. - Serve lunch

12:30 p.m. - Read, watch TV or movie, chat, and console whining patient

2:30 p.m. - Watch groggy patient sleep

3:30 p.m. - Play, talk, listen to endless patient health complaints

6:00 p.m. - Help get dinner together for picky-eater patient

6:30 p.m. - Sit in uncomfortable chair and keep grumpy patient happy

9:30 p.m. - Collect laundry, tuck in ungrateful patient, talk with nurses about patient's status

10:00 p.m. - Leave for home

10:30 p.m. - Eat something, read mail, start laundry, return phone calls

12:00 a.m. - Collapse into bed

I had a few touch-and-go evenings in the hospital over the past 14 years. On those occasions, M.G. either stayed all night or was there until 4:00 or 5:00 in the morning. Yikes! I'd rather be the patient.

Tip #120 Try to make your caregiver's job a little easier and less demanding whenever you can. If he or she looks exhausted, insist they leave for home earlier than usual and come in later the next day or take the day off.

Tip #121 Take responsibility for your own treatment. Never get snappy or short with a caregiver who's trying to keep you on track and get you back on your feet.

Tip #122 Refer to the Transplant Resource Directory for associations and organizations offering caregiver support, such as the National Family Caregivers Association, The Oncology Nursing Society, Support for Caring, and the Cancer Survivor Network.

Tip #123 Since hospital furniture is designed more for interrogations than for comfort, let your caregiver stretch out in the bed and you take the Geri chair.

Bonus Tip: Better yet, stretch out on the bed together and just try to breathe deeply and relax. It will work wonders.

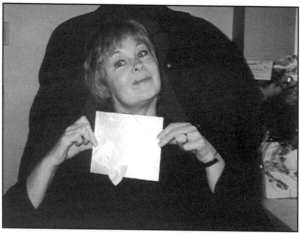

The ever-smiling M.G. at her post in the Geri chair.

Chapter 12

Keeping in Touch with Family and Friends

Almost every family has its political hierarchy. Siblings, parents, aunts, uncles, and cousins will often compete to be the first to find out anything new about your status or treatments so they can tell the others. This can be downright annoying.

The amount of time you spend communicating with your family depends, in large part, on how big your family is. I'm one of 10 children. M.G. is one of six. Throw in a half-dozen friends and you'd have to make the same phone call 20 times to bring everybody up to speed.

M.G. and I prefer the *Go it alone - Be left alone* approach. The reason for this is simple. Most of the time you're hospitalized, you're not going to feel like receiving visitors and making small talk. The many side effects from your treatment aren't conducive to partying. You'll quickly tire of people flopping on your bed, eating strange, smelly foods, bringing in things on the *Forbidden List*, and relentlessly asking you how you feel.

If you do have a *the more the merrier* personality, however, try to limit the number of visitors and the length of their stay so you don't wear yourself out.

Tip #124 M.G. set up a communication system that worked very well. She would call one person from each family every night, alternating people she called. She would ask that person to spread the news to the others. (This system is sometimes referred to as a telephone tree.) Viola! She only had to make 2 or 3 calls and everyone was in the loop.

Tip #125 Turn away anyone who is ill if they come to see you while you're neutropenic. Should there be any doubt regarding a visitor's health, have him or her wear a surgical mask.

Tip #126 Limit your visitors to a reasonable number. M.G. and I have seen transplant floors and patient lounges literally overrun with visitors gabbing, eating, talking on cell phones, using computers intended for patients, and generally being inconsiderate. Not cool.

Tip #127 Share the job of communicating with family and friends with your caregiver as soon as you're up to it. Make use of short e-mails and brief calls, no one really wants to hear all the gory details anyway.

Chapter 13

Being Discharged from the Hospital

It may seem like an eternity, but someday you'll get sprung from the hospital. Race home with a song in your heart, but keep an ever-watchful eye out for infections. You certainly don't want to wind up right back in the hospital.

Many transplant doctors like to get patients out of the hospital as soon as possible and send them home. Why? Because there's no better place to get sick than in a hospital.

The National Cancer Institute advises patients to be vigilant for the following symptoms of infection after being discharged:

- Fevers of over 100 degrees Fahrenheit
- Chills, especially if you have uncontrollable shaking (called the rigors)
- Sweating
- Loose bowel movements (can cause dehydration)
- Frequent urgency to urinate or burning with urination
- Sever cough or sore throat
- Unusual vaginal discharge

- Redness, swelling, or tenderness, especially around a wound, sore, ostomy, pimple, rectal area, or catheter site
- Sinus pain or pressure
- Earaches, headaches, or stiff neck
- Blisters on the lips or skin
- Mouth sores

Tip #128 Buy a thermometer for yourself as soon as you leave the hospital, if you don't already have one. Your temperature is an excellent indicator and rises whenever something bad is brewing. Immediately report any fever that climbs (spikes) to 100 degrees Fahrenheit or more.

Tip #129 Take your temperature a couple of times a day for a week or so to make sure you're OK It's almost impossible to tell if you have a fever if you're the one with the fever unless it's climbed very high.

Bonus Tip: Naturally, you'll be very anxious to leave the hospital when the time comes. Keep in mind, however, it's much more difficult to get assistance from doctors and nurses on the weekends. You might want to see if you can time your discharge for mid-week.

Bonus Tip: Every patient receives discharge instructions from the hospital. Follow them exactly.

Tip #130 Insurance companies would prefer you to be at home rather than in the transplant facility because it's cheaper. M.G. and I were sent home on one occasion to do an additional week of IV antibiotics. Stay in the hospital if you don't think you and your caregiver are up to sterilizing ports, lines, and connections; hanging IV bags; and starting and restarting the IV pump. M.G. did this three times a day for a week.

The majority of patients return to the center, their local hospital, or doctor's clinic to receive blood products and drugs in the weeks after they are released. Some blood products and drugs used to help patients until their counts recover are:

- Platelets (cells that keep you from bleeding)
- Red blood cells (cells that carry oxygen to your innards)
- G-CSF (a drug that stimulates white cell production)
- Procrit or Aranesp (drugs that stimulate the production of red blood cells

There are lots of other drugs you could be given, depending on your specific status. These include antibiotics, immunoglobulins (IVIG), antinausea drugs, pain medication, and a host of others.

Tip #131 You can plan the length of your follow-up stay based on the type of blood products you are scheduled to get. One unit of platelets takes about 20 to 30 minutes to infuse. A unit of red blood cells takes around two hours. It's not uncommon to have to be given several units of platelets or red blood cells in one session.

Tip #132 Some patients may have allergic reactions to infused blood products. Adverse reactions are fever, chills, hives, itching, shortness of breath, and heart palpitations (racing heart). Call you nurse immediately if you begin to experience any of these symptoms.

Bonus Tip (Men only): Resist the urge to play with the equipment when your nurse is out of the room. One day I thought my infusion was taking too long, so I turned the drip-rate up by myself. Within two minutes my left eye had swollen shut and my face was covered with hives. The nurses suggested duct taping my arms to the chair. M.G. told me, "See, Mark, bad things do happen to bad people."

Tip #133 Should you have an allergic reaction, the infusion will be stopped and you will be given something to counteract it, like steroids or Benedryl. Benedryl can make you very sleepy, so don't try to drive yourself home. Once your reaction is under control, the infusion will be restarted.

Chapter 14

Complementary and Alternative Medicine

Complementary and Alternative Medicine (CAM) has come out of the shadows in the past 20 years. Now, some of the most prestigious healthcare institutions in the country have CAM departments and protocols.

The National Institutes of Health defines CAM in the following manner: "Complementary and alternative medicine is a group of diverse medical and health care systems, practices, and products that are not presently considered to be part of conventional medicine.

Complementary medicine is used together with conventional medicine. An example of complementary therapy is using aromatherapy to help lessen a patient's discomfort following surgery.

Alternative medicine is used in place of conventional medicine. An example is using a special diet to treat cancer instead of undergoing surgery, radiation, or chemotherapy that has been recommended by a conventional doctor.

Integrative medicine combines mainstream medical therapies and CAM therapies for which there is some high-quality, scientific evidence of safety and effectiveness.

By some estimates, 50% of all cancer patients are using some form of CAM to augment their medical therapies."

The NIH lists five categories of CAM therapies on their Web site:

Alternative Medical Systems

1. Homeopathic medicine, naturopathic medicine, traditional Chinese medicine, and Ayurveda.

2. Mind-Body Interventions
   Visualization, meditation, prayer, mental healing, and creative therapies, such as art, music, and dance

3. Biology-Based Therapies
   Uses substance found in nature, like herbs, food, and vitamins and supplements many of which have yet to be proven scientifically

4. Manipulative and Body-Based Therapies
   Based upon manipulation and/or movement of one or more body parts including chiropractic and osteopathic manipulation and massage.

5. Energy Therapies
   Uses energy fields in two categories; biofield therapies and bioelectromagnetic-based therapies. Examples of the former are Qi gong, Reiki, and therapeutic touch. Examples of the latter are using pulsed fields, magnetic fields, or alternating or direct current fields.

Tip #134 Check with your doctor(s) before embarking on any of these CAM therapies.

Tip #135 Many CAM therapies have been proven safe and effective under normal circumstances. These are some your doc shouldn't have a problem with: support groups; massage therapy; music, art, and dance therapy, visualization, biofeedback, relaxation techniques, prayer, and meditation.

Tip #136 Some patients use visualization techniques, like imagining their new healthy stem cells are gobbling up any remaining cancer cells.

Bonus Tip: A study in the *Archives of Medicine* suggests prayer can be beneficial. CBSNews.com reported that researchers at the MidAmerica Heart Institute randomly divided 1,000 heart patients into two groups. The first group was prayed for daily. The second group was not. After four weeks, the prayed-for group had 10% fewer complications than the other group.

Bonus Tip: Be sure to tell your physicians and nurses if you are taking any kind of CAM medications. They may interfere with you prescription meds.

Chapter 15

Freebies for Transplantees

There are scads of free resources available from the associations and organizations listed in the Resource Directory in the next chapter. Here are some of the most valuable.

The American Cancer Society

www.cancer.org
800-ACS-2345
The ACS has 115 free brochures on just about every cancer topic. These can be reviewed online or ordered from the national or local office.

American Institute of Cancer Research

www.aicr.org
800-843-8114
Free 32-page brochure *CancerResource* can be read online or ordered by phone. Answers for many questions that arise after diagnosis.

BMT Infonet

bmtinfonet.org
800-597-7674
Free subscription to *The Blood & Marrow Transplant Newsletter.* Be sure to visit this site.

Gilda's Club

www.gildasclub.org
Provides free meeting places for men, women, and children living with cancer.

International Myeloma Foundation

www.myeloma.org

800-452-CURE

Visit this site or download a free copy of their booklet, *Autologous Bone Marrow and Stem Cell Transplantation* (Parts 1 & 2).

(The) Leukemia & Lymphoma Society

www.leukemia.org

800-955-4572

Has a free 68-page booklet entitled *Blood & Marrow Transplants.* Online library of over 300 articles on transplantation.

MEDLINEplus

www.medlineplus.org

Over 30 free articles on BMTs and PBSCTs.

Multiple Myeloma Research Foundation

www.multiplemyeloma.org

203-972-1250

Free, 40-page online booklet *Current and Emerging Trends in the Treatment of Multiple Myeloma.* It has an excellent section on transplantation.

National Bone Marrow Transplant Link

www.nbmtlink.org

800-546-5268

Offers four free booklets and one free video on the subjects of transplantation, including PBSCTs for breast cancer.

National Cancer Institute

www.cancer.gov

Provides 69 free publications some of which cover clinical trials, BMT and PBSCT Questions and Answers, self-help during chemotherapy, and pain relief.

National Coalition for Cancer Survivorship

www.canceradvocacy.org

877-622-7937

Has developed a free, comprehensive guide to living with cancer, *Essential Care*. Covers 12 aspects of survivorship.

Oncology Nursing Society

www.cancersymptoms.org

Free, online information about managing the six, common cancer treatment symptoms; fatigue, anorexia, pain, depression, neutropenia, and cognitive dysfunction.

The Bone Marrow Foundation

www.bonemarrow.org

212-838-3208

Read free booklets entitled *Allogeneic Bone Marrow and Stem Cell Transplantation* and *Autologous Bone Marrow and Stem Cell Transplantation*. Free online newsletter.

Chapter 16

Transplant Resource Directory

There's good news and bad news. The bad news, of course, is you or a loved one has cancer or some other debilitating illness. The good news, actually great news, is there's never been a better time to have cancer or other life-threatening diseases.

Survival rates are going up dramatically. Some estimate there are now over 9,000,000 cancer survivors in this country. Promising new treatments are being announced almost monthly. The amount of resources available to patients, families, and friends is truly amazing.

On the pages that follow, you'll find one of the most comprehensive resource directories ever compiled for those who are considering or are going to have a BMT or PBSCT.

If you don't have access to the Internet, try visiting your local library. Today, most libraries provide this service to patrons. The librarian or other staff members will help you get started if you've never used the Internet before. Can't get to the library? Call the organization you're interested in and they'll probably send the information you want free of charge. Most of the telephone numbers are toll-free. Many organizations or associations will have local chapters that can be found in the telephone book.

Please keep in mind, a listing in this resource section is not an endorsement of any kind. We are simply providing the information to assist you in making your own decisions. The claims made by the Web sites and organizations included are theirs, not ours. Also, Web sites simply promoting a single product such as a book or tape or program have not, as a rule, been included.

The more informed you are, the better your chances of enjoying a long and happy life. Be patient. Do your homework. Never stop learning.

About Cancer

www.cancer.about.com
Site offers top cancer books and videos, drugs
approved by the FDA, a guide to making treatment
decisions, and a database to search for doctors and
treatment centers.

AirLifeLine

www.airlifeline.org
877-AIR-LIFE
Coordinates free air travel for patients in need.

ALS Association

(amyotrophic lateral sclerosis)
www.alsa.org
818-880-9007

Alzheimer's Association

www.alz.org
800-272-3900

American Academy of Dermatology

(melanoma)
www.aad.org
888-462-DERM

American Brain Tumor Association

www.abta.org
800-886-2282

• American Cancer Society

www.cancer.org
800-ACS-2345
One of the absolute best sites for resources.
Information groups include: Learn about cancer;
treatment options; treatment decision tools; clinical
trials; and coping. Lots of stuff about BMTs and
PBSCTs. Really explore this site.

American Diabetes Association
www.diabetes.org
800-342-2383

American Foundation for
Urologic Diseases
(bladder, prostate, kidney cancers)
www.afud.org
800-242-2383

American Health and Healing
www.americanhealthandhealing.com
". . . we have created this wellness Web portal to
collect and organize the best wellness practices . . ."

American Institute for Cancer Research
www.aicr.org
800-843-8114
"AICR is the cancer charity that fosters research on
diet and cancer prevention and educates the public
about the results." Offers *A Resource Guide for those
Living with Cancer*, free online.

American Lung Association
www.lungusa.org
212-315-8700

American Sickle Cell Anemia Association
www.ascaa.org
216-229-4500

American Society of Clinical Oncology
www.asco.org
Great resources section. Covers: Patient Support
Organizations (tons); Cancer Centers & Cooperatives;
and Government Agencies.

- **Amgen**
  www.amgen.com
  Offers Neulasta and Neupogen (G-CSF). Also makes Palifermin to reduce severity of mucositis. Site provides patient information and links to additional resources.

- **Aplastic Anemia &
  MDS International Foundation**
  www.aplastic.org
  800-747-2820
  Foundation provides emotional support, educational materials, clinical trial listings, patient travel fund, and panel of experts.

  Asians for Miracle Marrow Matches
  www.asianmarrow.org
  888-236-4673

- **Association of Cancer Online Resources**
  www.acor.org
  Provides access to over 130 online communities (lists) for patients and families who need support. Communicate with people who have been in your spot.

- **Blood & Marrow Transplant
  Information Network**
  www.bmtinfonet.org
  888-597-7674
  "If a stem cell, bone marrow, or cord blood transplant is in your future, BMT Infonet can help." Has provided information and support to over 100,000 transplant patients since 1990. Sells books about transplants. Founder is a survivor who did a BMT in the early 1990s to treat leukemia (AML).

- **BMTnet**
  www.bmtnet.org
  "BMTnet is the new portal to blood and marrow transplantation resources on the World Wide Web." Provides links to blood and marrow transplant centers, meetings, and conferences.

- **BMT Support Online**
  www.bmtsupport.org
  586-575-9910
  "Our mission is to uphold those who suffer the effects of illness, before, during and after transplant . . ." Has online chat room for those who've had or are facing transplants.

Breast Cancer Recovery Foundation
www.bcrf.org

- **Cancer Federation**
  www.cancerfed.org
  The federation is a non-profit organization providing information, counseling, educational materials, and meetings for cancer patients, their families and friends.

Cancer Hope Network
www.cancerhopenetwork.org
877-HOPENET
"We match patients with trained volunteers who have themselves undergone a similar experience." Survivor stories.

- **Cancer Research and Prevention Foundation**
  www.preventcancer.org
  800-227-2732
  "Our mission is the prevention and early detection of cancer through scientific research and education." Offers *A Guide to Making Decisions About Your Cancer Therapy*, free online. Lists many resource links on their site.

Cancer Research Institute
  www.cancerresearch.org
  800-992-2623
  Click on Cancer HelpBook to find an 8-step program entitled *What to Do If Cancer Strikes*.

- **Cancer Survivors Network**
  www.acscsn.org
  800-ACS-2345
  Sponsored by the American Cancer Society. You can take advantage of *Talk Shows & Stories,* start your own, personal Web page, join in discussions and chats, and share your interests and experiences with other survivors.

- **CancerCare**
  www.cancercare.org
  Offers information on drug assistance programs, financial assistance, finding home care, finding hospice care, and finding transportation. Describes Hill-Burton Program, which can arrange for free or low cost care. Also outlines the AVONCares Program. Very good site.

- **CancerEducation.com**

  www.cancereducation.com

  212-531-5960

  Site has *MedClip* streaming audio lectures you can watch. Contains information on drugs, finding a physician, and finding a treatment center.

- **Cancerfacts.com**

  www.cancerfacts.com

  "This online resource for cancer patients, their families, and caregivers is dedicated to delivering accurate and personalized information at a time of need. The NexProfiler™ Tools for Cancer help people with cancer make informed treatment decisions for an optimal outcome."

- **CancerGuide**

  www.cancerguide.org

  CancerGuide was started by a fellow survivor. The site has material on clinical trials, survivors stories, how to use medical libraries, rare cancers, and BMTs.

CancerHelp

www.cancerhelp.8m.com

Has links to Web sites that deal with specific types of cancers. Good online resources list. There are mailing lists and support groups.

- **CancerIndex**

  www.cancerindex.org

  "This site contains over 100 pages and more than 4,000 links to cancer-related information." Has a first-rate glossary of cancer words and terms.

CancerLinks
www.cancerlinks.com
510-649-8177

CancerNews
www.cancernews.com
"Dedicated to bring patients and their families the latest news and information on cancer diagnosis, treatment, and prevention.

• Cancerpage
www.cancerpage.com
Detailed material on BMTs and PBSCTs. Offers chat rooms and support groups.

CancerQuest
www.cancerquest.org
This site, sponsored by Emory University, was "created to teach the biology of cancer." Could be too technical for many.

• CancerSource.com
www.cancersource.com
617-399-4483
This site provides live chat events, message boards, mailing lists, support groups, online cancer drug database, treatment information, clinical trial data, and a cancer dictionary.

Cancervive
www.cancervive.org
800-4-TO-CURE
"Dedicated to providing support, public education, and advocacy to those who experience this disease." You can share your story here.

Candlelighters Childhood Cancer Foundation
www.candlelighters.org
800-366-2223
"A national, non-profit membership organization whose mission is to educate, support, serve, and advocate for families of children with cancer, survivors of childhood cancer, and the professionals who serve them."

• **Coalition of Cancer Cooperative Groups**
www.cancertrialshelp.org
877-520-4457
"Our mission is to increase survival and improve the quality of life of cancer patients through increased participation in cancer clinical trials." Offers *TrialCheck* to help visitors determine trial eligibility and location.

Coping with Cancer Magazine
www.copingmag.com
"Now in its 17th year of providing knowledge, hope, and inspiration . . ."

Corporate Angel Network
www.corpangelnetwork.org
866-328-1313
"We arrange for free air transportation for cancer patients traveling to treatment centers using empty seats on corporate jets."

Cure Magazine
www.curetoday.com
800-210-CURE
"Cancer Updates, Research, and Education is a quarterly magazine that combines the science and humanity of cancer for those who have to deal with it on a daily basis." Offers free subscription.

Cycle of Hope
(Lance Armstrong Foundation)
www.cycleofhope.org
512-236-8820
"Shows how learning facts will lessen your fears, help you regain control of your emotions, and ultimately increase your chances of beating cancer."

Gilda's Club Worldwide
www.gildasclub.org
888-GILDA-4-U
". . . to provide meeting places where men, women, and children living with cancer and their family and friends can join with others to build emotional and social support."

Headcovers Unlimited
www.headcovers.com
580-226-5871
Sells hats, turbans, hats with hair, scarves, sleep hats, wigs, toupees, eyebrows and eyelashes.

Health Insurance Information
www.healthinsuranceinfo.net
Offers a publication entitled *A Consumer Guide for Getting and Keeping Health Insurance* for every state.

Hospice Education Institute
www.hospiceworld.com
800-331-1620
"HEI serves a wide range of individuals and organizations interested in improving and expanding hospice and palliative care . . ."

- **Immune Deficiency Foundation**
www. primaryimmune.org
800-296-4433
Go to this Web site and click on the heading
Publications. From this page, click on *Specific Medical Therapy*. You'll find an extensive, online document about BMTS and PBSCTs.

International Cancer Alliance for Research and Education
www.icare.org
800-ICARE61
This site posts *Clinical Therapy Reviews* for over 40 types of cancer. Also has Clinical Trials Matching Program.

- **International Myeloma Foundation**
www.myeloma.org
800-452-CURE
Visit this site and get a free copy of their booklet, *Autologus Bone Marrow and Stem Cell Transplantation,* parts 1 & 2. Offers free Myeloma Info Pack.

Kidney Cancer Association
www.kidneycancerassociation.org
800-850-9132

Kidscope
www.kidscope.org
404-892-1437
"One of our goals is to help children successfully cope with the diagnosis and treatment of a parent with cancer."

Lance Armstrong Foundation
www.laf.org
512-236-8820
"LAF exists to enhance the quality of life for those living with and beyond cancer."

Look Good . . . Feel Better
www.lookgoodfeelbetter.org
800-395-LOOK
"LGFB is a free, non-medical, national public service program to help women (and teens) offset appearance-related changes from cancer treatment."

Lupus Foundation of America
www.lupus.org
202-349-1155

Lymphoma Information Network
www.lymphomainfo.net
"Your comprehensive guide to Hodgkin's and Non-Hodgkin's Lymphoma." Features books, videos, survivor stories, and a glossary.

• Lymphoma Research Foundation
www.lymphoma.org
800-235-6848
Site offers a 1-hour, online audio visual presentation on allogeneic and autologus transplants.

MD Anderson Cancer Center
www.mdanderson.org
800-392-1611
Gives visitors an opportunity to search clinical trials. Type the word transplants in the search box.

Make-A-Wish Foundation
www.wish.org
800-722-WISH
Grants the wishes of children with life-threatening
medical conditions to enrich the human experience
with hope, strength and joy.

MAMM
www.mamm.com
A magazine devoted to meeting the needs of women
diagnosed with breast and reproductive cancer.

• MEDLINEplus
(Part of the National Institutes of Health)
www.medlineplus.org
Click on the *Health Topics* tab. Next, click on the
Procedures & Therapies heading and select the
subheading *Bone Marrow Transplantation*. That will
bring up over 30 articles on BMTs and PBSCTs.
Articles cover topics such as transplant basics, Q&A
about transplantation, choosing a provider, and facts
and figures.

Memorial Sloan-Kettering Cancer Center
www.mskcc.org
212-639-2000
Once at the site, select the *Transplantation* tab to find
thorough information.

Multiple Myeloma Association
www.webspawner.com/users/myelomaexchange
Has detailed information on leading cancer centers
treating myeloma. These centers do thousands of
transplants a year. Has a discussion list.

- **Multiple Myeloma Research Foundation**
www.multiplemyeloma.org
203-972-1250
Site offers a free, 40-page online booklet, *Current and Emerging Trends in the Treatment of Multiple Myeloma*. It has a very good section on transplantation.
(Go you fellow myelomians!)

- **National Bone Marrow Transplant Link**
www.nbmtlink.org
800-LINK-BMT
You can get a free copy of *A Resource Guide For Bone Marrow/Stem Cell Transplant - Friends Helping Friends*. This document provides details on financial aid, insurance, pediatric transplantation, and selecting a caregiver.

- **National Cancer Institute**
(Part of the National Institutes of Health)
www.cancer.gov
800-4-CANCER
From the home page, click on *Cancer Information*, then click *Treatment*, and click *Types of Treatment*. *Select BMT and PBSCT Questions and Answers*.

National Center for Complementary and Alternative Medicine
(Part of the National Institutes of Health)
www.nccam.nih.gov
888-644-6226
Here, you can review articles on understanding complementary and alternative medicine, research, and clinical trials.

- **National Comprehensive Cancer Network**
www.nccn.org
"The NCCN, an alliance of 19 of the world's leading cancer centers, is an authoritative source of information to help patients and health professionals make informed decisions about cancer care."

National Foundation for Transplants
www.transplants.org
800-489-3863 ext. 101
"Organ and bone marrow transplant patients nationwide turn to NFT when they need help in raising funds for transplant costs not covered by insurance."

- **National Institutes of Health**
www.health.nih.gov
Excellent documents on transplants, clinical trials database, resource information, and drug information. NIH has over 40 toll-free information lines for specific diseases and conditions. Plan to spend a lot of time at this site.

- **National Marrow Donor Program**
www.marrow.org
800-MARROW2
"The NMDP helps people who need a life-saving marrow or cord blood transplant. We connect patients, doctors, donors and researchers to resources they need to help more people live longer, healthier lives." Has facilitated over 15,000 unrelated donor transplants.

National Multiple Sclerosis Society
www.nmss.org

National Ovarian Cancer Coalition
www.ovarian.com
888-OVARIAN

National Parkinson Foundation
www.parkinson.org

Native American Cancer Research
www.members.aol.natamcan
303-838-9359

Needy Meds
www.needymeds.com
215-625-9609
"Many drug manufacturers have what's called Patient Assistance Programs. These programs are designed to help those who can't afford their medicines obtain them at no cost or low cost." Site contains information on over 200 drug company programs.

Nueva Vida
www.nueva-vida.org
202-223-9100
"The mission of Nueva Vida is to inform, support, educate, and empower Latinas affected by cancer, and to advocate for and facilitate the timely access to state of the art cancer care . . ."

OncoLink
www.oncolink.org
215-349-5445
Offers an *Ask the Expert* feature whereby patients, family, or friends can pose questions to oncologists.

Oncology Nursing Society

www.cancersymptoms.org
Provides information on learning about and managing each of six common cancer treatment symptoms; fatigue, anorexia, pain, depression, neutropenia, and cognitive dysfunction.

Ontumor.com

www.ontumor.com
Lots of resources for newly diagnosed cancer patients.

Pancreatic Cancer Action Network

www.pancan.org
877-272-6226

Patients Against Lymphoma

www.lymphomation.org
Provides "Evidence-based resources for patients and professionals, independent of health industry funding." Offers free online brochures and tools.

• People Living with Cancer

www.peoplelivingwithcancer.org
"Provides oncologist approved information on more than 50 types of cancer and their treatments, clinical trials, coping, and side effects. Also includes live chats, message board, drug database, medical dictionary, and links to patient support organizations."

• Pharmaceuticals Research and Manufacturers Association

www.helpingpatients.org
Sponsored by PhRMA and 48 member companies to help find patient assistance programs for medicines.

R.A. Bloch Cancer Foundation
www.blochcancer.org
Features on this site include: 12 questions to ask your doctor, patient's checklist for fighting cancer, Positive Mental Attitude quiz, and the ability to be matched to a volunteer who has the same type of cancer.

Sarcoma Foundation of America
www.curesarcoma.org
301-520-7648
Key the word *transplant* into the search box for a survivor story.

Sisters Network
www.sistersnetworkinc.org
"It is our mission to increase local and national attention to the devastating impact that breast cancer has on the African American community.

Susan G. Komen Breast Cancer Foundation
www.komen.org
Breast Care Helpline: 800-I'M Aware
The foundation is a global leader in the fight against breast cancer. Provides valuable resources for patients, survivors, and affiliates. Online message board.

• The Bone Marrow Foundation
www.bonemarrow.org
212-838-3208
"We hope this site will provide you with the resources, information, programs and services about bone marrow/stem cell transplantation you need whether you are a patient, family member, friend, bone marrow donor or health care professional."

- **The Cancer Information Network**
  www.thecancer.info
  "The Network is founded on the belief that proactive patients who educate themselves to take an active role in decisions about their therapy can effect their outcomes in a positive way."

- **The Leukemia & Lymphoma Society**
  www.leukemia.org
  800-955-4572
  Search the word *transplants* here and you can review more than 300 articles. Offers a free, 68-page online booklet, *Blood and Marrow Transplants*, with a glossary. Too many services to list. Visit or call. Offers financial assistance.

  The Mautner Project for Lesbians with Cancer
  www.mautnerproject.org
  Offers support groups, bereavement groups, survivor workshops, and a national Peer Support Network.

- **The Myelodysplastic Syndromes Foundation, Inc.**
  www.mds-foundation.org
  Devoted to the prevention, treatment and study of myelodysplastic syndromes. Lists MDS Centers of Excellence. Search for MDS clinical trials at this site.

- **The Wellness Community**
  www.thewellnesscommunity.org
  Offers professionally led support groups, educational workshops and mind/body programs utilizing the Patient Active Concept.

United States Department of Health and Human Services
(Health Resources and Services Admin.)
www.hrsa.gov/osp/dot/choosebmt.htm
Has an online document called *Considerations for Choosing a Bone Marrow Transplant Provider.* Contains over 30 points to consider when selecting a provider for your transplant.

WebMD
www.webmd.org
Key the words *stem cell transplants* into the search box at this site and you'll get over 70 professional articles on the subject. Well worth the time to sift through them to find what you need.

• **Sites of particular interest for transplant patients.**